Maintaining Diet

by

Nathan R.kinne

Maintaining Diet

Table of contents

Chapter 2

Menu for the future (Malnutrition results from shy salutary input)

. <u>Vitamins</u>

. <u>Mineral</u>

. <u>Protein</u>

. Fat

. Carbohydrate (sugar)

.Water

Chapter 3

Consume healthy food

. Why is vital to eat healthy

. Advantage of eating well

. Among the consequence inadequate nutrition are:

Chapter 4

How to lose weight and keep it off

The Diabetes Diet

What about the glycemic indicator?

Conclusions

Maintaining Diet

Introduction: Maintaining Your Diet shows readers how adding the right foods to your diet can reduce harmful body fat, stop your body from breaking down, and help you lose weight in a way that will extend your life and improve your overall health.

You must maintain a sufficient and sustainable calorie deficit in order to lose weight. You must make sure you're getting enough calories and protein in order to develop healthy muscle mass.

Making sure you're getting the right kinds and amounts of carbohydrates at the right times is essential for optimal athletic performance.

You can get a good idea of what's entering your body by keeping track of the food you eat. This implies that you'll be able to make wiser decisions and get the most out of your exercise regimen.

Maintaining your diet will allow you to see exactly what you're putting into your body. This implies that you'll be able to make wiser decisions and get the most out of your exercise regimen. You remain a human being despite not adhering to strict body composition guidelines or having competitive objectives.A diet is the total amount of food that an individual or other organism eats.The term "diet" frequently connotes the application of a particular dietary intake for weight-management or health-related purposes (the two are frequently connected). Despite the fact that all people are omnivores, different cultures and individuals have different dietary preferences and taboos. This could be for moral or taste-related reasons. A person's food choices may or may not be healthful.

You're still a human being even if you don't follow rigid body composition guidelines or pursue competitive objectives. Understanding how to fuel your body will help you make the most of

it,feel the best about it, and extend its life.

If you are trying to reach a goal, you can see where you can improve if you are also keeping track of your calories. You can use it to determine whether you are eating too little or too much.

Maintaining Diet

Chapter 1

Calculating calories

Weight loss is the term used to describe a decrease in total body weight. Aside from underlying medical issues, there are additional causes of weight loss. A few examples include starvation, exercise, diets, and restricted food access. A common goal that many people have had for a long time is to reduce their body fat and weight. Not only are gaining muscle mass and decreasing weight appealing aesthetic objectives, but they are also critical steps in improving our general health. In weight loss regimens that support health and decrease cholesterol and blood pressure, burning calories is essential.

Weight loss is inevitable when you eat less than your body needs. To put it another way, eat less and move more. It will tap your body in this manner.

A huge reduction on the scale can give us the boost and motivation that we need.Because it will provide you with the energy you need in the morning, breakfast has the potential to be one of the most important meals of the day to kickstart your metabolism.Fat loss only covers weight loss from fat, but weight loss from stored carbohydrates, protein, water, and fat might also be included.Fat loss typically occurs at a slower rate. Like most individuals, you probably want to know as soon as possible after starting your weight loss journey when you may anticipate seeing results. Simultaneously, you could also be interested in finding out if the weight you're reducing is coming from fat or muscle.

Why is weight loss necessary for some people?

An individual who is overweight has an increased chance of contracting potentially fatal diseases. Being overweight may make you more susceptible to type 2 diabetes and several types of cancer. Additionally, there is an increased risk of gallstones, infertility, sleep apnea, heart disease, and high blood pressure. Those who are overweight should be sufficiently motivated to change their habits and way of life under these circumstances. Losing weight can improve the physical and mental well-being of those who suffer from depression, low self-esteem, and humiliation.

What leads to obesity and a rise in weight?

Genetics may be contributing factors to obesity

instances, particularly when a child is born to obese parents. Of course, a major factor in determining which genes express themselves and which do not is what is consumed.

Processed foods can be addicting and contain additives and processed components. By carefully positioning products in supermarkets to make unhealthy food seem attractive and by advertising low pricing and bargains, the manufacturers of these products actively encourage overeating. They advertise bad foods as healthy in certain unethical ways.

A *lot* of sugar-filled foods are frequently linked to narcotics, alcohol, and nicotine in terms of how they affect the brain, leading to addiction, overindulgence, and intense desires for junk food.

When overindulged, foods high in sugar can alter the body's biochemistry and hormones.

How can one avoid gaining weight?

Adopting a healthy lifestyle that involves regular physical activity and better eating habits can help avoid weight gain. Selecting healthful and nutrient-dense foods such fruits, vegetables, fish, lean meats, and legumes should be the aim.

Eating little and frequently throughout the day and including these foods into the diet to "crowd out" unhealthy processed meals like refined carbs and foods high in sugar is a good strategy. When exercise is incorporated into a regular practise, weight loss and calorie burning are potential outcomes.

Phases of losing weight

. Quick drop of weight You generally lose the most weight during the first stage of weight loss, which is also when you start to notice changes in your appearance and apparel fit. generally, it occurs in the first four to six weeks. At this point, the main causes of weight loss are water, protein, and glycogen reserves; body fat accounts for a lower portion of the weight reduction. People who follow low- carb diets tend to lose weight briskly than those who follow low- fat diets because they use up their body's carbohydrate and water coffers more snappily. But if a low- carb or ketogenic diet is better than a low- fat diet in the long run for total weight reduction rudiments other than diet, including your age, coitus, starting weight, and physical exertion position, can also impact your rate of weight loss.

For illustration, men are more likely to lose weight

hastily than women, and aged grown-ups may lose weight hastily than their youngish counterparts, although some of this weight loss may be muscle. On the other hand, if you start out heavier and exercise more regularly, you will presumably lose weight briskly.

How to lose weight in some simple way (losing weight is a choice one must make to achieve a positive result)

1. Consume fat, vegetables, andprotein.Every mess should aim to point a range of foods. refections should have a balance of complex carbohydrates, fat, protein, and vegetables on your plate. Eating a recommended quantum of protein is essential to help save muscle mass while losing Diets with acceptable protein may also reduce Trusted Source jones and snacks by helping you feel full and satisfied.

2. Good fats Nuts, seeds, avocados, olive oil painting, and other healthy fats are excellent additions to your diet. Keep in mind that canvases are made entirely of good fats. While some — like olive oil painting — are regarded as healthy, they also have a advanced calorie content per gramme at nine, as opposed to four for protein and carbohydrates. Because of this, it's critical to consume good fats in temperance and to minimise trans and

impregnated fats. Fat loss simply involves weight reduction from fat, albeit slipping pounds can also include smaller pounds through protein, water, fat, and carbohydrates that have been accumulated. Loss of fat generally happens more sluggishly. Like utmost individualities, you presumably want to know as soon as possible after starting your hunt to lose weight about the time you may anticipate seeing results. contemporaneously, you could also be interested in chancing out if the weight you are reducing is coming from fat or muscle.

The stages of weight loss, the distinction between fat loss and weight loss, and strategies for avoiding weight gain are all covered in this composition.

Loss of weight generally happens in two stage

AN ORIGINAL, QUICK STAGE & a POSTERIOR, SLOWER, MORE PROLONGED STAGE.

Stage 1.Food instability may affect from extended weight loss. Not getting enough nutrients in your diet can lead to malnutrition. Those who suffer from digestive diseases like celiac complaint, which impact the body's capability to absorb nutrients, may find this to be particularly true.

Stage 2.Slow weight reduction The alternate stage of

weight loss is significantly slower to develop and substantially results from body fat; this stage generally lasts longer than sixweeks.Because of metabolic adaptations that lower your metabolism and the quantum of calories you burn when exercising, you may sometimes witness a weight loss table during which you lose little to no weight. But the reason weight loss mesas more constantly be is that a lot of diets are extremely delicate to stick to and too rigid, which leads to individualities sinning fromthem.So that you can maintain it over time, it's critical to cleave to a salutary plan that suits your preferences and way of life.

Why is loosing weight vital for some humans?

An individual who is overweight has an increased chance of contracting potentially fatal diseases. Being overweight may make you more susceptible to type 2 diabetes and several types of cancer. Additionally, there is an increased risk of gallstones, infertility, insomnia, heart disease, alongside elevated levels of cholesterol. Those who are overweight ought to be sufficiently motivated to change their habits and way of life by these circumstances. Losing weight can improve the physical and mental well-being of those who suffer from depression, low self-esteem, and humiliation.

How can one avoid gaining weight?

Adopting a healthy lifestyle that involves regular physical activity and better eating habits can help avoid weight gain. Selecting healthful and nutrient-dense foods such as fruits, vegetables, fish, lean meats, and legumes should be the aim.Eating little and frequently throughout the day and including these foods in the diet to "crowd out" unhealthy processed meals like refined carbs and foods high in sugar is a good strategy. When exercise is incorporated into a daily habit, calories will be burned, and weight loss is probably possible.

OVERVIEW

There are two stages to weight loss: a quick weight loss phase and a delayed

weight loss phase. You'll see the biggest physical changes during the quick weight loss period.

Maintaining Diet

CHAPTER 2

Menu for the future (Malnutrition results from shy salutary input)

The biochemical and physiological process through which an organism uses food to sustain itself is known as nutrition. It gives organisms nutrients that they can metabolise to produce chemical structures and energy. The process of ingesting food and turning it into energy and other essential factors demanded for life is known as nutrition. The kind of paraphernalia known as nutrients give the body the energy and biomolecules it needs to perform a variety of tasks. While all living goods in the creation bear nutrients for healthy growth and operation, there are differences in the ways that these conditions are met. Malnutrition, or nutrient crunches, be when an organism does not have enough of any given nutrient. The biochemical and physiological process through which an organism uses food to sustain itself is known as nutrition. It gives organisms nutrients that they can metabolise to produce chemical structures and energy. The process of ingesting food and turning it into energy and other essential factors demanded for life is known as

.Nutrition

The kind of paraphernalia known as nutrients give the body the energy and biomolecules it needs to perform a variety of tasks. While all living goods in the creation bear nutrients for healthy growth and operation, there are differences in the ways that these conditions are met. Malnutrition, or nutrient crunches, be when an organism does not have enough of any given nutrient. similar to how spare can be dangerous. One of the numerous goods that bring all people together, despite our differences, is eating. To live, we must each eat. We sometimes bear backing choosing what to eat and when. People fight in some corridor of the world to consume enough food, and in other corridor, they battle to eat too important. also there are those who struggle greatly to eat the food necessary for their quotidian conditions and others who bear backing in making opinions that will cover their health. Vitamins, minerals, protein, lipids, water, and carbs are the six nutrients that are demanded. These nutrients must be attained via diet for people's bodies to serve duly. These nutrients must be attained via diet for people's bodies to serve properly. Essential nutrients are necessary for a person's growth, health, and reduplication. The two types of these necessary nutrients are called macronutrients and micronutrients.

Micronutrients are substances that the body need in trace quantities. Minerals and vitamins are samples of micronutrients. The body only requires trace quantities of these, but a insufficiency might have negative health goods. A person need macronutrients in lower quantities. Water, protein, carbs, vitamins, minerals, and lipids are samples of macronutrients. It's important to flash back that there are six orders of necessary nutrients vitamins, minerals, protein, fats, water, and carbohydrates. These nutrients must be attained via diet for people's bodies to serve duly.

.Vitamins

An existent should acquire cornucopia of vitamins from a diet high in fruits, vegetables, and healthy meat. Micronutrients called vitamins have a number of health advantages, analogous as strengthening the vulnerable system could help defer or avoid some malignancy, analogous prostate cancer bolstering bones and teeth, easing the immersion of calcium, conserving skin health, and abetting the body's metabolism of protein and carbohydrate sources maintaining respectable blood flux to the brain and neurological system Nutritionists classify the thirteen essential vitamins under two groups water answerable and fat answerable. Vitamins answerable in fat are vitamins D and A vitamins K and E The following vitamins are water answerable thiamine(vitamin B- 1) and cyanocobalamin(vitamin B- 12). B- 6 vitamin the B- 2 vitamin riboflavin Pantothenic acid, or vitamin B- 5, Niacin, or vitamin B- 3, vitamin B- 9(folic acid and folate) Biotin, or vitamin B- 7, and vitamin C A person eating a diet high in fruits, vegetables, and spare proteins may generally gain all the vitamins they bear from their refections. To lessen or help a insufficiency, people with digestive issues and those who consume lower fruits and vegetables may need to take a vitamin supplement.

.**Minerals**:

The alternate class of micronutrients is minerals. Major and trace minerals are the two orders of minerals. For optimum health, the body need a balance of minerals from both orders. pivotal minerals are phosphorous, sulphur, magnesium, calcium, sodium, potassium, and chloride The following functions of the organism are backed by major minerals water equilibrium. keep your nails, hair, and skin healthy. strengthen your bones Mineral traces are metal iron, zinc, and manganese, Chromium, bobby , fluoride, iodine, and molybdenum

Among the benefits of trace minerals are stronger bones. avoiding dental caries. helping the blood to clot. carrying oxygen in the process. abetting the defence medium. promoting blood pressure that is good You can make sure you eat enough minerals by include these foods in your diet. red flesh(use them sparingly and handpick spare cuts) shellfish, dairy products, and iodized table tar(lower than 2,300 mg daily). seeds and nuts vegetable crisp flora berries chuck and cereals amended with flesh egg whites whole grains legumes and sap Dietetics and Nutrition.

.Protein

Each and every cell in the body requires protein as a macronutrient in order to operate correctly. There are numerous places that proteins perform. dependable force, analogous as guaranteeing the conformation of hormones, antibodies, and other necessary composites that act as a energy source for cells and apkins when demanded, as well as the growth and development of skin, muscles, bones, hair, and other apkins. Through their diet, you can consume proteins. Good sources of protein include the following foods red flesh; handpick spare cuts and use them sparingly. fish and other seafood, as well as fowl, analogous as funk and lemon leguminous shops ovaries dairy goods. nuts made from soy Certain grains, analogous as quinoa Insectivores and insectivores can gain respectable protein from a variety of factory particulars, indeed though flesh and fish generally have the topmost protein content.

.Fat

Foods high in fat are constantly linked to poor health. But in order to help sustain optimum health, a person requires specific fats. The body uses fats for energy and to perform a variety of other tasks. But it's vital to eat lipids that are good for you, analogous as mono- and polyunsaturated fats, and to minimise or stay down from trans and saturated fats. Good fats support the following processes cell division blood coagulation and cell division lowering the chance of type 2 diabetes and heart complaint, muscle movement, and blood glucose brain exertion immersion of vitamins and minerals hormone conflation immunological response Good fats can be set up in a variety of foods, analogous as nuts, seeds, vegetable canvases , and seafood like tuna and salmon.

Carbohydrate(sugar)

The body needs carbohydrates for proper function. All of the body's apkins and cells get their energy from these sugars, also known as beans. Carbohydrates come in two kinds simple and complicated. Rice, spaghetti, and white chuck

 are exemplifications of simple carbs that people should consume in temperance. still, the following functions of the organism arestem digestion process According to the Dietary Guidelines, a person should get 45 – 65 of their quotidian energy from complex carbs. The foods listed below are rich in complex carbohydrates Quinoa. brown rice with veggies chuck , spaghetti, and other baked particulars made with whole grains cereal, fruits, and barley White flour that has been blanched and reused exorbitantly, as well as dishes with fresh.

.Water

Probably the most vital nutrient that humans require is water. It takes a while for an individual to go without water. Dehydration, even mild cases, can lead to headaches and poor physical and mental performance.

Water accounts up the majority of the human body, and water is necessary for every cell to operate. Water aids in a number of processes, such as removing pollutants, absorbing shock, carrying nutrients, and avoiding constipation.

Hydration and lubrication

Water from the tap or bottles is the best source of natural, unsweetened water. People who dislike the flavour of plain water can add other citrus fruits or a dash of lemon.

Fruits that are high in water content can also provide an additional source of water for a person.

 Sugary drinks should not be consumed in place of the recommended daily water intake.

Fruit juices, soda, coffee, teas with added sugar, and lemonade are examples of sugary beverages.The study of dietetics focuses on how food and nutrition impact human health. The study of dietetics places a high priority on public health and is dedicated to informing people about the value of making healthy food decisions.Nutritionists who specialise in dietetics use food science and nutrition to help individuals become healthier. In order to care for and counsel patients, nutrition and dietetic technologists collaborate with dieticians and nutritionists. General nutrition education can also be given by nutrition and dietetic technicians as well as dietitian nutritionists.The process of taking in, absorbing, and putting to use the nutrients that the body needs for development, growth, and life maintenance is known as nutrition.People need to eat a balanced diet that includes a variety of nutrients—the compounds in foods that nourish the body—in order to acquire adequate, optimal nutrition.

Maintaining Diet

Chapter 3

Consume healthy food

Eating a nutritious diet has numerous advantages; it affects not only your bodily but also your mental and emotional well-being. For this reason, the Broken Plate 2022 annual report from the Food Foundation raises a lot of concerns.

If current trends continue, almost 80% of 2022-born children who live to be 65 years old will be overweight or obese. Of them, at least one in twenty will have passed away already.

In only the last year, there has been a 50% increase in childhood obesity. Obesity in children increases the risk of diet-related disorders in adulthood. Obesity has a negative impact on one's physical and mental well-being, self-esteem, and academic performance.

Growth retardation is a result of poor nutrition. Five-year-olds in Britain are shorter than those in the European counterparts, and there is a significant disparity in height between affluent and impoverished regions of the nation.

The number of life-limiting amputations brought on by

diabetes-related problems associated with obesity has reached all-time highs, dramatically lowering the quality of life for those afflicted and putting a tremendous strain on both our healthcare system and the general economy.

The cost of nutrient-dense, healthful food is over three times that of obesogenic, unhealthy goods; an equivalent quantity of 1,000 calories of more nutritious meals costs an average of £8.51, whereas less nutritious items only cost £3.25.

Every time, the UK incurs direct NHS charges of nearly£ 74 billion due to redundant weight, together with lost productivity from the pool and docked life expectation. The 20- time difference in healthy life expectation between the flush and poorest parts of society is substantially due to it. Eating a range of foods that give you with the nutrients you need to feel good about yourself, have energy, and save your health is considered healthy eating. Consuming a nutritional diet does not have to be delicate or confining, and you do not have to give up your favourite foods. Balance is the key. For our bodies and minds to remain healthy, we all bear a varied and well- balanced diet rich in protein, fat, carbs, fibre, vitamins, and minerals. also, we must maintain portion balance, which entails eating the applicable quantities of food for our bodies. Unhealthy weight and physical issues can affect from gorging and inactivity. Undereating in order to make up for the energy we use can also affect in malnutrition, unhealthy weight, and physical affections. The thing of healthy eating is to choose the healthiest options available in each food order and, whenever doable, to substitute natural foods for reused bones

. Foods containing meliorated grains, like meliorated wheat or white flour, have high bounce content, which the body simply stores rather than using. Make an trouble to consume further whole grains, similar as oats, brown rice, and wholewheat chuck

, foods like brown rice, oats, and the suchlike, which give you energy for a longer time after eating them. Making good eating choices is pivotal if you want to eat healthily. This goes for both refections and snacks.

Why is it vital to eat healthily?

A nutritional diet is essential for overall well- being. It's imperative to guard you against multitudinous habitualnon-communicable ails, including cancer, diabetes, and heart complaint. The nutrients in the food you eat support diurnal conditioning, shield your cells from detriment from the terrain, and help repair any implicit damage to your cells. Because your gut is so important to your digestion and metabolism, it's pivotal to support the health of your gut with a proper diet and life. Its main jobs include breaking down and absorbing food as well as barring waste. On the other hand, your gut produces 90 of the serotonin in your body. Serotonin is a neurotransmitter that travels throughout your body and between brain cells to convey dispatches. It's essential for maintaining bone health, blood coagulation, crack mending, mood, sleep, digestion, nausea, and sexual desire, among other fleshly processes. An poor, out- of- balance diet can negatively affect your physical and emotional health as well as your intestinal health. tutoring kiddies to eat healthy foods from an early age is also pivotal. Healthy eating promotes a child's physical and internal growth as well as their capability to concentrate and stay energetic, all of which support a child's capability to study throughout the academy day. Healthy eating habits and preferences are formed beforehand on and remain that way for the rest of one's life. styles for Eating Well A healthy diet can not be specified in a one- size- fits- all manner; nevertheless, the main effects to keep in mind are to consume an cornucopia of fruits and vegetables, whole grains, and spare protein sources like fish or beats, while cutting back on reused foods, sugar, and alcohol. You can make numerous simple salutary adaptations to ameliorate its health; these correspond of Eating breakfast energies your body and helps you start the day off right. Eat smaller refections throughout the day. Rather than consuming a big lunch and regale, try eating lower amounts more constantly. circumscribe your input of sticky foods and potables as they can spike and fall blood sugar situations, lead to tooth decay, and raise rotundity. Snack on fruit rather of sticky foods like galettes, chocolate, and biscuits. To stay doused , exchange out sticky drinks for water or water- grounded potables and aim to consume six to eight spectacles of fluid daily. Eat lower red meat Although red meat, similar as beef, overeater, or angel, is a healthy source of protein, eating too much of it can raise your threat of heart complaint and high cholesterol.

Because they are heavy in saturated fat, try limiting or avoiding processed meats like sausages and burgers.

Eat a serving of oily fish each week. Omega-3 fatty acids, which are abundant in oily fish like salmon and trout, are excellent for heart health and can reduce your chance of developing heart disease.

Eat five times a day. Vitamins, minerals, and other elements that are essential for immune system support and overall health are abundant in fruits and vegetables.

Eat an abundance of legumes. Peas, beans, and lentils are all low in fat, high in protein, and a fantastic way to add bulk to meals.

Create meals that revolve around foods high in fibre. Eating a diet high in fibre helps lower your risk of heart disease, high blood pressure, type 2 diabetes, and high cholesterol. Select wholegrain or wholemeal bread, rice, and pasta as they are higher in fibre, vitamins, and minerals than white ones.

Incorporate dairy or dairy substitutes into your diet. Products like milk, yoghurt, and cheese are high in calcium, which helps maintain healthy bones and teeth and can stave off osteoporosis as you age. This can also be obtained from fortified dairy substitutes like oat milk or soy products, along with a variety of other vitamins and minerals.

 Anything with trans fats or partially hydrogenated oils listed on the label should be avoided, as they both boost bad cholesterol and lower good cholesterol.

Advantage of eating well

Healthy eating has a lot of advantages.Consuming a nutritious diet will guarantee your continued health for a long time while giving you the energy and nutrition you need to stay active throughout the day.Reduce your chance of developing long-term illnesses like heart disease, type 2 diabetes, and some types of cancer.bolster the immune system.assist in the digestive system's operation.assist in keeping a healthy weight.Maintain strong, healthy bones and teeth.bolster and repair muscle.Boost your energy levels.Encourage the health and function of the brain.Improve mood. assistance with sleeping habits.

Encourage children's healthy development and growth.

Encourage wholesome pregnancies.

Among the consequences of inadequate nutrition are:

Obesity: An unhealthy diet high in fat and sugar can lead to obesity, which is a significant risk factor for a number of illnesses.

High cholesterol: High cholesterol can result in major health issues including constricted blood arteries.

High blood pressure, sometimes referred to as hypertension, can result from eating a bad diet and, if unchecked, can cause heart failure, strokes, and renal disease.

Diabetes: A diet heavy in fat, carbs, sugar, and cholesterol, along with being overweight and sedentary, are risk factors for type 2 diabetes.

Cancer: Studies indicate that eating a diet low in nutrients may raise your chance of getting some malignancies, like colon cancer.

Bone loss - An inadequate diet deficient in calcium and vitamin D can raise your risk of osteoporosis, a disorder that weakens and fractures bones.

Heart disease and stroke: High blood pressure and cholesterol are two additional diet-related health issues that can raise your risk of heart disease and stroke.

Mental health and mood A dip in blood sugar can cause fatigue, irritability, and depression.

Essentials of a nutritious diet

The World Health Organisation (WHO) and the Food and Agriculture Organisation (FAO) of the United Nations (FAO) concur on the essentials of a healthy diet.

These tenets are To make sure you are getting enough nutrients, eat a range of refections. Consume a lot of fruits and veggies. at least 400g, or roughly five servings, of fruits and vegetables each day. Eat nuts, whole grains, and unsaturated fats to maintain a healthy diet. Limit your consumption of impregnated fats. impregnated fats should make up lower than 10 of total sweet input in grown-ups to avoid noxious weight gain. Consume lower sugar. For farther health benefits, limit your input of free sugars to lower than 10 or 5 of your overall energy. This translates to 50g or 25g of free sugars daily, consequently. Reduce the quantum of swab. One tablespoon, or lower than five grammes, of swab each day. Regularly belt water. Staying well doused is essential for good health. drinking of alcohol. Alcohol isn't a element of a healthy diet because there's no safe quantum to consume it at. Reference inputs(RI) are recommendations for the approximate volume of specific nutrients and energy demanded for a diet that promotes health. These are guidelines, determined by the government, that indicate the recommended diurnal input of each nutrient for a healthy average person. RIs are an effective tool to help us understand food and make healthier opinions on a diurnal base, indeed though eating a balanced and varied diet is still the most important thing to do. RIs are grounded on a typical lady who's at a healthy weight, has no specific salutary requirements, and engages in moderate exercise. You should use the calorie RI as a reference. The maximum recommended inputs for fat, impregnated fat, sugar, and swab are the RIs. RIs are present on food markers and give nutritive data for each portion grounded on a chance of the RIs. 8400 kJ/ 2000 kcal of energy. lower than 70 grammes of total fat. lower than 20g is satisfying. Minimum of 260g of carbohydrates. 90g of total sugars. 50g protein. lower than 6g of swab. Eating well while celiac In the UK, one in every 100 people has celiac complaint. When you ingest gluten, it can beget a dangerous sickness where your body assaults its own apkins with the vulnerable system. A balanced and healthy diet must include fibre. Because entire grains like wheat, rye, and barley are barred from a gluten-free diet, it may be poor in fibre. Brown rice is one type of whole grain that's free of gluten. popcorn among sludge. Amaretti. Warm wheat. Oats devoid of gluten. emmet. Lettucc. Soybean. It's estimated that 25 of adult cases with celiac complaint are anaemic as a result of iron insufficiency at opinion. Iron from shops isn't as well absorbed as iron from creatures. Red meat is a good source of iron that's applicable for a gluten-free diet. still, because of its high vitamin A content, liver and liver products should be avoided by pregnant women. eggwhite.green veggies withleaves.pulses like lentils, sap, andpeas.dried fruit, including figs, raisins, andapricots.Seeds andnuts.Individuals who suffer from celiac complaint can bear further calcium than the average adult population. At least 1,000 mg of calcium should be consumed daily by grown-ups with celiac complaint. 700 mg is the suggested lozenge for the generalpublic.Semi- skimmed milk is a good source of calcium that's applicable for a gluten-freediet.soy milk enhanced withcalcium.Sardines in a can with bones cheesecheddar.yoghurt.Kale.Bakedlegumes.renalbeans.Walnuts.cauliflower.preserved apricots. Eating well while lactose intolerant Around 68 of people on the earth experience the symptoms of indecorous lactose digestion, which is caused by milk sugar. Although it's constantly mistaken for a milk mislike, lactose dogmatism isn't an mislike. Steering clear of utmost, but not all, dairy particulars that may beget issues is common while avoiding lactose. It's pivotal to make sure you're entering enough of the vitamins and minerals you would generally find in dairy products because they're significant sources of calcium, protein, and vitamins A, B12, andD. Several excellentnon-dairy calcium sources include Non-dairy milks and fruit authorities have redundant calcium in them. Wholegrain cereals and tofu with added nutrients can also help you get the calcium you need. Hard crapola with low to no lactose content include cheddar and parmesan. Sardines and anchovies, among other fish with small, comestible bones, are rich in calcium. Calcium is set up in dark leafy vegetables including kale, chard and collard flora. still, you can be dairy-free and yet maintain acceptable calcium situations, If you eat balanced refections and incorporate foods high in calcium into your diet. Insectivores' healthy eating habits It's generally believed that eating a vegan diet lowers your threat of heart complaint, high blood pressure, high cholesterol, and type 2 diabetes. In addition to cutting out meat and fish from their diets, insectivores also hesitate from all foods deduced from creatures, including dairy, eggs, and honey. also, they don't include specific E figures, similar as the red food colouring cochineal(E120), rennet, which is used to make rubbish, or gelatine, which is used in goodies. Some submissive dishes, like some meat druthers, are banned from the menu due to their egg and sometimes dairy content. Because they consume so numerous fruits and vegetables, vegan diets are high in fibre, vitamin C, and folate. still, they may be deficient in other vitamins and minerals, like as vitamin B12. Because vitamin B12 is typically set up in beast foods like eggs, milk, and rubbish, insectivores must make sure their diets include enough of it by include fortified breakfast cereals, soy products, and incentive excerpt. Vitamin B12 is necessary for healthy red blood cells and neurological function. Iron may be set up in shops, and insectivores can enhance their input of this vital mineral by consuming factory- grounded foods together with high- vitamin C foods like citrus fruits and peppers. Making main courses out of legumes, sap, and tofu will guarantee that a vegan diet doesn't lack protein.

Vegan diets tend to be low in saturated fat, but they may also be deficient in heart-healthy kinds of omega-3 fats, which are typically found in shellfish and fish. Nuts, seeds, and their oils, along with specific micro-algae supplements and sea vegetables like kelp, can all be beneficial. Healthy skin and hair can be preserved with the help of lipids derived from cold-pressed hemp, rapeseed, walnut, or flaxseed oil.

Vegans must make sure that any supplements they take, including extra vitamins, are suitable for vegan diets.

Last reflections on

These are the fundamental components of a nutritious, well-balanced diet, and there are several ways to combine them depending on our own nutritional needs, tastes, and cultures.

Since each person is unique, the guidelines for a healthy diet can be modified to fit your needs. Since food is designed to be enjoyed, it is totally possible to eat the things you love and still nourish your body healthily.

Maintaining Diet

Chapter 4

How to Lose Weight and Keep It Off

There's a better way to lose weight. These gorging tips can help you avoid diet pitfalls and achieve lasting weight- loss success. What's the swish diet for healthy weight loss? So, what should you believe? The verity is there is no " one size fits all " affect to endless healthy weight loss. To find the system of weight loss that's right for you will presumably take time and bear forbearance, commitment, and some trial with different foods and diets. While some people respond well to counting calories or similar restrictive styles, others respond better to having farther freedom in planning their weight- loss programs. So, don't get too discouraged if a diet that worked for notoriety else doesn't work for you. . Flash back while there's no easy fix to losing weight, there are cornucopia of way you can take to develop a healthier relationship with food, check emotional triggers to gorging, and achieve a healthy weight.

Four popular weight loss

1. Cut calories Some experts believe that successfully

managing your weight comes down to a simple equation If you eat lower calories than you burn, you lose weight. Sounds easy, right also.

why is losing weight so hard?

Weight loss isn't a direct event over time. When you cut calories, you may drop weight for the first numerous weeks, for illustration, and also commodity changes. You eat the same number of calories but you lose lower weight or no weight at all. That's because when you lose weight you're losing water and spare kerchief as well as fat, your metabolism slows, and your body changes in other ways. So, A calorie isn't always a calorie. Eating 100 calories of high fructose sludge sentimentality, for illustration, can have a different effect on your body than eating 100 calories of broccoli. The trick for sustained weight loss is to gutter the foods that are packed with calories but don't make you feel full(like delicacy) and replace them with foods . multitudinous of us don't always eat simply to satisfy hunger. We also turn to food for comfort or to relieve stress which can snappily

unhinge any weight loss plan for comfort or to relieve stress which can snappily unhinge any weight loss plan.

2. Cut carbs. A different way of viewing weight loss

identifies the problem as not one of consuming too multitudinous calories, but rather the way the body accumulates fat after consuming carbohydrates in particular the part of the hormone insulin. When you eat a mess, carbohydrates from the food enter your bloodstream as glucose. In order to keep your blood sugar situations in check, your body always burns off this glucose before it burns off fat from a mess. still, rice, chuck , If you eat a carbohydrate-rich mess(lots of pasta. As well as regulating blood sugar situations, insulin does two goods It prevents your fat cells from releasing fat for the body to burn as energy(because its priority . The result is that you gain weight and your body now requires farther energy to burn, so you eat more. To lose weight, the sense goes, you need to break this cycle by reducing carbs. utmost low- carb diets plump replacing carbs with protein and fat, which could have some negative long- term goods onyourhealth.However, you can reduce your risks and limit your input of saturated and trans fats by choosing spare meat, fish and amenable sources of protein, If you do try a low- carb diet.

3. Cut fat. It's a dependence of multitudinous diets if you don't want to get fat, don't eat fat. Walk down any grocery store aisle and you'll be bombarded with

reduced- fat snacks, dairy, and packaged refections. So,

why haven't low- fat diets worked for further of us?

Not all fat is bad. Healthy or " good " fats can actually help to control your weight, as well as manage your moods and fight fatigue. Unsaturated fats set up in avocados, nuts, seeds, soy milk, tofu, and adipose fish can help fill you up, while adding a little succulent olive oil painting oil to a plate of vegetables, for illustration, can make it easier to eat healthy food and meliorate the overall quality of your diet.

We frequently make the wrong trade- offs. numerous of us make the mistake of switching fat for the empty calories of sugar and meliorated carbohydrates. rather of eating whole- fat yoghurt, for illustration, we eat low- or no- fat performances that are packed with sugar to make up for the loss of taste. Or we change our adipose breakfast bacon for a muffin or donut that causes rapid fire harpoons in blood sugar.

4. Follow the Mediterranean diet The Mediterranean diet emphasizes eating good fats and good carbs along with large amounts of fresh fruits and vegetables, nuts, fish,

and olive oil painting — and only modest quantities of meat and rubbish. The Mediterranean diet is further than just about food, however. Regular physical exertion and sharing refections with others are also major factors. . Do you eat when you are upset, wearied, or lonely? Do you snack in front of the television at the end of a stressful day? . If you eat when you're Stressed – find healthier ways to calm yourself. Try yoga, contemplation, or soaking in a hot bath. Low on energy – discovery other mid - afternoon pick- me- ups. Try walking around the block, harkening to amping music, or taking a short nap. Lonely or wearied – reach out to others rather of reaching for the refrigerator. Call a friend who makes you laugh, take your canine for a walk, or go to the library, boardwalk, or demesne — anywhere there is people. Practice aware eating rather Avoid distractions while eating. Try not to eat while working, watching television, or driving. It's too easy to mindlessly gourmandize Pay attention. Eat sluggishly, savoring the smells and textures of yourfood.However, gently return your attention to your food and how it tastes, If your mind wanders. Mix effects up to concentrate on the experience of eating. Try using tablewares rather than a chopstick, or use your implements with predominant hand. Stop eating before you're full. Do not feel indebted to always clean your plate. Ways to Reduce Weight and Maintain It Losing weight can be done more effectively. You can achieve long- term weight loss success and steer clear of diet problems by using these overeating guidelines.

What's the ideal diet to lose weight in a healthy way?

Take any diet book and it'll promise to give you with all the results you need to successfully lose all the weight you want and keep it off. Some say that the secret is to eat lower and exercise more; others suppose that eating low fat is the sole option; still others advise giving up carbohydrates. And so,

what are you to believe?

The fact is that sustainable, healthy weight loss can not be achieved with a" one size fits each" approach. Because our systems reply else to different refections grounded on genetics and other health considerations, what works for one person might not work for you. Chancing the stylish weight reduction plan for you'll presumably take some time, tolerance, fidelity, and some experimenting with colorful foods and diets. While counting calories or other restrictive strategies work effectively for some people, giving them further latitude to design their weight- loss programmes works more for others. Allowing children to simply hesitate from fried refections or reduce their input of refined carbohydrates can place them for success. thus, if a diet that has worked for someone differently does not work for you, do not give up tooquickly.In the end, a diet is only good for you if it's commodity you can maintain over time. Recall that although reaching a healthy weight is delicate, there are numerous effects you can do to ameliorate your relationship with food, reduce the emotional triggers that lead to gluttony, and cultivate a positive relationship with food. Four well- liked diet programmes Reduce the number of calories. Some experts suppose that controlling your weight can be boiled down to this straightforward formula you lose weight if you consume smaller calories than you burn. It seems simple enough.

Why is weight loss so delicate?

Losing weight isn't a gradational, direct process. For illustration, during the first two weeks of cutting calories, you may lose weight, but after that, commodity changes. Indeed though you consume the same quantum of calories, you either gain no weight at all or lose veritably little. This is due to the fact that weight loss causes your body to change in other ways, decelerate down your metabolism, and beget you to lose fat in addition to water. therefore, you must keep reducing your sweet input if you want to continue losing weight each week. Not every calorie is the same as the coming. For case, your body may rcply else to 100 calories of broccoli than it may to 100 calories of high fructose sludge saccharinity. Foods grandly in calories but low in satisfaction, similar as delicacy, should be avoided in favour of calorie- thick, satisfying foods, similar as vegetables, if you want to lose weight over time. Not everyone eat only to fill the bellies.Additionally, we turn to food for solace or stress relief, which can fleetly throw off any weight loss programme. for ease or as a way to relax — which can fleetly throw off any weight- loss strategy. Lower carbs An indispensable perspective on weight loss attributes the problem to the body's process of storing fat following carbohydrate consumption, specifically the function of the hormone insulin, rather than an excess of calories consumed. During a mess, the food's carbohydrates are convcrtcd to glucose in your bloodstream. Your body always uses up this glucose before burning fat after a mess to maintain healthy blood sugar situations. Your body releases insulin in response to eating a mess high in carbohydrates, similar as French feasts, pasta, rice, or chuck , to help your blood absorb all of the glucose. In addition to controlling blood sugar, insulin also prevents fat cells from releasing fat for the body to burn as energy (since the body's first precedence is to burn off glucose) and promotes the growth of new fat cells to store any redundant fat that the body is unfit to burn off. You gain weight as a result, which makes you eat more because your body needs further energy to burn it. You get into a vicious cycle of eating carbohydrates and gaining weight because insulin only burns carbohydrates, which makes you crave them. The thinking goes that cutting carbs is the key to breaking this cycle and losingweight.The maturity of low- carb diets recommend substituting fat and protein for carbohydrates, which may have some unfavourable long- term healtheffects.However, you can lower your input of trans and impregnated fats and minimise your threat by consuming plenitude of lush green andnon-starchy vegetables, low- fat dairy products, If you choose to try a low- carb diet.

Trim fat.A common diet tenet is to avoid eating fat if you want to gain weight. Reduced- fat snacks, dairy products, and prepackaged refections will be thrown at you whenever you tromp down any grocery store aisle. still, as the number of low- fat foods has increased, so too have rotundity rates.

Why have not further people set up success with low-fat diets?

Fat isn't always bad. In fact, " good" or healthy fats can fight fatigue, regulate your mood, and help you maintain a healthy weight. Avocados, nuts, seeds, soy milk, tofu, and adipose fish are rich sources of unsaturated fats that can fill you up. also, spraying some succulent olive oil painting over a plate of veggies can grease the consumption of healthy foods and enhance the flavour of the food. frequently, we choose the incorrect trade-offs.A common mistake made by numerous of us is to replace empty calories from sugar and meliorated carbohydrates with fat. For illustration, we eat low- or no- fat performances of yoghurt that are loaded with sugar to make up for the taste loss rather than whole- fat kinds. Alternately, we replace our adipose bacon for a muffin or donut that harpoons our blood sugar snappily for breakfast. Borrow a Mediterranean eating style.

The Mediterranean diet places a strong emphasis on consuming plenitude of fresh fruits and vegetables, nuts, fish, and olive oil painting, as well as healthy fats and carbohydrates. Meat and rubbish are only relatively consumed. But the Mediterranean diet is about further than just food. Other important Rudiments include eating refections together and engaging in regular physical exertion. Anyhow of the weight loss plan you choose, it's critical to maintain provocation and steer clear of typical gluttonousness risks like emotional eating. Reduce your emotional eating. Not all of the time do we eat to satisfy our hunger. When we are upset or stressed-out- eschewal- eschewal- eschewal- avoidance, we tend to turn to food each too constantly, which can ruin any diet and beget weight gain

When you are anxious, jaded, or lonely, do you eat?

Do you relax with a snack in front of the television after a demanding day? If you consume food while Feeling stressed-out? Look for healthier ways de-stress. Indulge in a hot bath, yoga, or contemplation.

Feeling sluggish?

Look for indispensable instigations. Try going for a quick perambulation around the block, putting on some upbeat music, or taking a quick nap. Reach out to people when you are wearied or lonely, rather than opening the fridge. Go for a walk with your canine, make a call to a friend who makes you laugh, or visit any public place where people congregate, like a demesne or library. rather, engage in aware eating. When eating, stay down from distractions. Avoid eating when operating a vehicle, watching television, or working. It's too simple to overeat without allowing. Bc aware. Savour the flavours and textures of your food as you eatslowly.However, gently bring them back to the flavour of your food, If your studies slideshow. To put the emphasis on the eating experience, mix effects up. rather of using a chopstick, try using tablewares, or use predominant hand to handle your implements. Eat until you're satisfied. Your brain needs some time to admit the signal that you've had enough. You do not have to clear your plate every time. Stay inspired. Make healthy salutary and life adaptations for long- term weight loss. To remain inspired Slow and steady wins the race. Losing weight excessively nippy can take a trouble on your mind and body, making you feel sluggish, drained, and sick. Set pretensions to keep you motivated. Short- term pretensions, like wanting to fit into a bikini for the summer, generally do not work as well as wanting to feel more confident or come healthier for your children's sakes. Use tools to track your progress. Get cornucopia of sleep. Lack of sleep stimulates your appetite so you want further food than normal; at the same time, it stops you feeling satisfied, making you want to keep eating. Sleep privation can also affect your provocation, so aim for eight hours of quality sleep a night. Cut down on sugar and perfected carbs Whether or not you are specifically aiming to cut carbs, ultimate of us consume unhealthy quantities of sugar and perfected carbohydrates similar as white chuck, pizza dough, pasta, afters, white flour, white rice, and candied breakfast cereals. Replacing perfected carbs with their whole- grain counterparts and barring delicacy and delectables is only part of the result, still. Sugar is hidden in foods as different as canned mists and vegetables, pasta sauce, margarine, and numerous reduced fat foods. Since your body gets each it needs from sugar naturally being in food, all this added sugar quantities to nothing but a lot of empty calories and unhealthy harpoons in your blood glucose. lower sugar can mean a slimmer midriff Calories attained from fructose(set up in sticky potables similar as soda pop pop pop and reused foods like doughnuts, muffins, and delicacy) Cutting back on sticky foods can mean a slimmer midriff as well as a lower trouble of diabetes. Fill up with fruit, veggies, and fiber Indeed if you are cutting calories, that does not inescapably mean you have to eat lower food. High- fiber foods similar as fruit, vegetables, tire, and whole grains are advanced in volume and take longer to digest, making them filling and great for weight- loss. It's generally okay to eat as important fresh fruit annunciation vegetables as you want — you'll feel full before you've bloated it on the calories. Eat vegetables raw or fumed, not fried or breaded, and dress them with gravies and spices or a little olive oil painting oil oil painting for flavor. Add fruit to low sugar cereal — blueberries, strawberries, sliced bananas. You will still enjoy lots of agreeableness, but with lower calories, lower sugar, and further fiber. Snack on carrots or celery with hummus rather of a high- calorie chips and dip. Add further veggies to your favourites main courses to make your dish more substantial. Indeed pasta and stir- feasts can be diet- friendly if you use lower polls and further vegetables. Start your mess with salad or vegetable haze to help fill you up so you eat lower of your entrée. Take charge of your food terrain Set yourself up for weight- loss success by taking charge of your food terrain when you eat, how important you eat, and what foods you make fluently available. Cook your own refections at home. Restaurant and packaged foods generally contain a lot further sugar, unhealthy fat, and calories than food cooked at home plus the portion sizes tend to be larger. Serve yourself lower portions. Use small plates, colosseums, and mugs to make your portions appear larger. Do not eat out of large colosseums or directly from food holders, which makes it delicate to assess how important you've eaten.

Eat Beforehand

Studies suggest that consuming further of your quotidian calories at breakfast and lower at regale can help you drop more pounds. Eating a larger, healthy breakfast can jump- start your metabolism, stop you feeling empty during the day, and give you farther time to burn off the calories. Fast for 14 hours a day. Try to eat regale ahead in the day and also presto until breakfast the coming morning. Eating only when you're most active and giving your digestion a long break may prop weight loss. You can produce your own small portion snacks in plastic bags or holders. Eating on a schedule will help you avoid eating when you aren't truly empty. Drink further water. Thirst can constantly be confused with hunger, so by drinking water you can avoid spare calories. Limit the amount of tempting foods you have athome.However, store indulgent foods out of sight, If you partake a kitchen withnon- swillers. Exercise can increase your metabolism and meliorate your outlook and it's commodity you can benefit from right now. Go for a walk, stretch, move around and you'll have farther energy and provocation to attack the other way in your weight- loss program. Lack time for a long drill? Three 10- minute spurts of exercise per day can be just as good as one 30- nanosecond drill. Flash back anything is better than nothing. Start off slowly with small amounts of physical exertion each day. also, as you start to lose weight and have farther energy, you'll find it easier to come more physically active. Find exercise you enjoy. Try walking with a friend, dancing, hiking, cycling, playing Frisbee with a canine, enjoying a blitz game of basketball, or playing exertion- rested video games with your youths. Keeping the weight off You may have heard the extensively quoted statistic that 95 of people who lose weight on a diet will regain it within a numerous times or indeed months. While there's n't much hard evidence to support that claim, it's true that multitudinous weight- loss plans fail in the long term. constantly that's simply because diets that are too restrictive are truly hard to maintain over time. still, that does n't mean your weight loss attempts are doomed to failure. Far from it. Since it was established in 1994, The National Weight Control Registry(NWCR) in the United States, has tracked over 10,000 individualities who have lost significant amounts of weight and kept it off for long periods of time. Whatever diet you use to lose weight in the first place, espousing these habits may help you to keep it off Stay physically active. Successful gorgers in the NWCR study exercise for about 60 beats, generally walking. Keep a food log. Recording what you eat every day helps to keep you responsible and motivated. Eat breakfast every day. utmost generally in the study, it's cereal and fruit. Eating breakfast boosts metabolism and staves off hunger subsequently in the day. Eat further fiber and lower unhealthy fat than the typical American diet. Regularly check the scale. importing yourself daily may help you to descry any small earnings in weight, enabling you to directly take corrective action before the problem escalates. Watch lower television. Cutting back on the time spent sitting in front of a screen can be a vital part of espousing a more active life and preventing weight gain.

The Diabetes Diet

Healthy eating can help you help, control, and indeed

hamper diabetes. And with these tips, you can still enjoy your food without feeling empty or deprived. What is the swish diet for diabetes? Whether you are trying to help or control diabetes, your nutritive conditions are nearly the same as everyone differently, so no special foods are necessary. But you do need to pay attention to some of your food choices most especially the carbohydrates you eat. Losing just 5 to 10 of your total weight can help you lower your blood sugar, blood pressure, and cholesterol situations. Losing weight and eating healthier can also have a profound effect on your mood, energy, and sense of good. People with diabetes have nearly double the trouble of heart complaint and are at a lower trouble of developing internal health conditions similar as depression. But utmost cases of type 2 diabetes are preventable and some can indeed be reversed. Indeed if you 've formerly developed diabetes, it's not too late to make a positive change. By eating healthier, being further physically active, and losing weight, you can reduce your symptoms. Taking way to help or control diabetes docs n't mean living in privation; it means eating a succulent, balanced diet that will also boost your energy and ameliorate your mood. You do n't have to give up sweets entirely or abnegate yourself to a continuance of mellow food. The biggest trouble for diabetes belly fat Being fat or fat is the biggest trouble factor for type 2 diabetes. still, your trouble is advanced if you tend to carry your weight around your gut as opposed to your hips and knives. A lot of belly fat surrounds the abdominal organs and liver and is nearly linked to insulin resistance. You're at an increased trouble of developing diabetes if you are A woman with a midriff circumference of 35 elevation or further A man with a midriff circumference of 40 elevation or further Calories attained from fructose(set up in sticky potables similar as soda pop pop pop, energy and sports drinks, coffee drinks, and reused foods like doughnuts, muffins, cereal, delicacy and granola bars) are more likely to add weight around your gut Cutting back on sticky foods can mean a slimmer midriff as well as a lower trouble of diabetes. The first step to making smarter choices is to separate the myths from the data about eating to help or control diabetes.

Myths and data about diabetes and diet Myth You must avoid sugar at all costs. Fact You can enjoy your favorite treats as long as you plan duly and limit retired sugars. Cate does not have to be off limits, as long as it's a part of a healthy mess plan. Fact The type of carbohydrates you eat as well as serving size is vital. Focus on whole grain ca rbs rather of stiff carbs since they are high in fiber and digested sluggishly, keeping blood sugar situations more indeed. Myth You will need special diabetic refections. precious diabetic foods generally offer no special benefit. Myth A high- protein diet is voguish. Fact Studies have shown that eating too important protein, especially beast protein, may actually beget insulin resistance, a vital factor in diabetes. Our bodies need all three to serve duly. The key is a balanced diet. As with any healthy eating program, a diabetic diet is further about your overall salutary pattern rather than obsessing over specific foods. Aim to eat more natural, undressed food and lower packaged and convenience foods. Eat further Healthy fats from nuts, olive oil painting oil canvas , fish oil paintings, flax seeds, or avocados. Fruits and vegetables immaculately fresh, the further various the more; whole fruit rather than authorities. High- fiber cereals and victuals made from whole grains. Fish and shellfish, organic funk or lemon. High- quality protein similar as eggs, tire, low- fat dairy, and thin yogurt. Eat lower Packaged and presto foods, especially those high in sugar, burned goods, sweets, chips, delectables. White chuck sticky cereals, perfected pastas or rice. Reused meat and red meat. Low- fat products that have replaced fat with added sugar, similar as fat-free yogurt. Choose high- fiber, slow- release carbs Carbohydrates have a big impact on your blood sugar situations more so than fats and proteins so you need to be smart about what types of carbs you eat. Limit perfected carbohydrates like white chuck pasta, and rice, as well as soda pop pop pop, delicacy, packaged refections, and snack foods. Focus on high- fiber complex carbohydrates also known as slow- release carbs. They're digested more sluggishly, therefore precluding your body from producing too important insulin.

What about the glycemic indicator?

High glycemic indicator(GI) foods spike your blood sugar fleetly, while low GI foods have the least effect on blood sugar. While the GI has long been promoted as a tool to help manage blood sugar, there are some notable downsides. Having to relate to GI tables makes eating unnecessarily complicated. exploration suggests that by simply following the guidelines of the Mediterranean or other heart-healthy diets, you will not only lower your glycemic weight but also ameliorate the quality of your diet. smart about sweets Eating a diabetic diet oesn't mean barring sugar altogether, but like ultimate of us, chances are you consume further sugar than is healthy. Still, you can still enjoy a small serving of your favourites cate now and also, If you have diabetes. The key is temperance. Reduce your acceptance for sweets by sluggishly reducing the sugar in your diet a little at a time to give your taste youths time to acclimate. Hold the chuck(or rice or pasta) if you want delicacy Eating sweets at a mess adds spare carbohydrates so cut back on the other carb-heavy foods at the same mess. Add some healthy fat to your delicacy Fat slows down the digestive process, meaning blood sugar situations do not spike as snappily. That does not mean you should reach for the donuts, still. suppose healthy fats, similar as peanut adulation, ricotta rubbish, yogurt, or nuts. Eat sweets with a mess, rather than as a stage-alone snack. When eaten on their own, sweets beget your blood sugar to shaft. But if you eat them along with other healthy foods as part of your mess, your blood sugar will not rise as fleetly. When you eat delicacy, truly savory each bite. How numerous times have you mindlessly eaten your way through a bag of babes or a huge piece of galette?. You will enjoy it more, plus you are less likely to gormandize. Tricks for cutting down on sugar Reduce soft drinks, soda pop pop pop, and juice. For each 12 oz. serving of a sugar- candied drink you drink a day, your trouble for diabetes increases by about 15. Try foamy water with a twist of bomb or lime rather. Do not replace impregnated fat with sugar. numerous of us replace impregnated fat similar as whole milk dairy with refined carbs, allowing we are making a healthier choice.. Candy foods yourself. Buy thin iced tea, plain yogurt, or unflavored oatmeal, for illustration, and add sweetener(or fruit) yourself. You will presumably add far less sugar than the manufacturer. Check markers and conclude for low sugar products and use fresh or frozen constituents rather of canned goods. Be especially alive of the sugar content of cereals and sticky drinks. Avoid reused or packaged foods like canned mists, concrete feasts, or low- fat refections that constantly contain retired sugar. Prepare further refections at home. Reduce the quantum of sugar in fashions by

¼ to ⅓. You can boost agreeableness with mint, cinnamon, nutmeg, or vanilla excerpt rather of sugar. rather of ice cream, blend up frozen bananas for a delicate, frozen treat. Or enjoy a small clump of dark chocolate, rather than a milk chocolate bar. Start with half of the food you generally eat, and replace the other half with fruit. Be And combinations mixed with soda pop pop pop and juice can be loaded with sugar. Choose calorie-free mixers, drink only with food, and cover your blood glucose as alcohol can intrude with diabetes drug and insulin.

living sharp about sweets is only part of the battle of reducing sugar and simple carbs in your diet. Sugar is also hidden in multitudinous packaged foods, fast food refections, and grocery store millions analogous as chuck , cereals, canned goods, pasta sauce, margarine, instant mashed potatoes, concrete feasts, low- fat refections, and ketchup. Sugar is also hidden in multitudinous packaged foods, fast food refections, and grocery store millions analogous as chuck, cereals, canned goods, pasta sauce, margarine, instant mashed potatoes, concrete feasts, low- fat refections, and ketchup. The first step is to spot sheltered sugar on food labels, which can take some sleuthing Manufacturers give the total amount of sugar on their labels but do not have to separate between added sugar and sugar that is naturally in the food. Added sugars are listed in the ingredients but are n't always easily recognizable as analogous. While sugar, honey, or molasses are easy enough to spot, added sugar could also be listed as sludge sweetener, high- fructose sludge sentimentality, faded club juice, agave drinkable, club dishes, invert sugar, or any kind of fructose, dextrose, lactose, maltose, or sentimentality. While you 'd anticipate sticky foods to have sugar listed near the top of their list of ingredients, manufacturers constantly use different types of added sugars which also appear scattered down the list. But all these little pilules of different sweeteners can add up to a lot of spare sugar and empty calories!Overall, choose good fats, including unsaturated fats and saturated fats from a variety of vegetables, nuts, seeds, fish and undressed meat. Avoid bad fats analogous as partly hydrogenated oils and saturated fats in reused meat.(saturated) fats. set up mainly in tropical oils, red meat, and dairy, there's no need to completely count logged fat from your diet but rather, enjoy in temperance. The American Diabetes Association recommends consuming no further than 10 of your quotidian calories from saturated fat. Healthy(unsaturated) fats. The healthiest fats are unsaturated fats, which come from fish and plant sources analogous as olive oil painting oil oil p ainting oil painting oil, nuts, and avocados. Omega- 3 adipose acids fight inflammation and support brain and heart health. Good sources include salmon, tuna, and flaxseeds.

Ways to reduce unhealthy fats and add healthy fats rather of chips or crackers, snack on nuts or seeds or add them to your morning cereal. Nut adulation are also truly satisfying. rather of frying, choose to melee, sear, or stir- bash. Avoid saturated fat from reused meat, packaged refections, and takeout food. rather of just red meat, vary your diet with skinless funk, eggs, fish, and amenable sources of protein. Use extra - abecedarian olive oil painting oil oil painting oil painting oil to dress salads, cooked vegetables, or pasta dishes. marketable salad dressings are constantly high in calories so produce your own with olive oil painting oil oil painting oil painting oil, flaxseed oil painting oil oil painting oil painting oil, or sesame oil painting oil oil painting oil painting oil. Along with being loaded with healthy fats, they make for a filling and satisfying mess. Enjoy dairy in temperance. Eat regularly and keep a food journal It's encouraging to know that you only have to lose 7 of your body weight to cut your trouble of diabetes in half. Eat at regularly set times Your body is better suitable to regulate blood sugar situations and your weight when you maintain a regular mess schedule. Aim for moderate and harmonious portion sizes for each mess.. It will give energy as well as steady blood sugar situations. Eat regular small refections — over to 6 per day.. Keep calorie input the same. To regulate blood sugar situations, try to eat roughly the same amount every day, rather than gorging one day or at one mess, and also pinching the coming. Keep a food journal A recent study set up that people who kept a food journal lost twice as important weight as those who didn't. Why? A written record helps you identify problem areas analogous as your afterlife snack or your morning latte where you're getting farther calories than you realized. It also increases your awareness of what, why, and how important you're eating, which helps you cut back on careless snacking. Keep a tablet handy or use an app to track your eating. Get more active Exercise can help you manage your weight and may meliorate your insulin perceptivity. An easy way to start exercising is to walk for 30 beats a day(or for three 10- minute sessions if that's easier). You can also try swimming, biking, or any other moderate- intensity exertion that has you working up a light sweat and breathing harder. multitudinous individualities have formed habits when it comes to eating. There are some that are healthier than others(" I always have fruit for cate"), like" I always have a sticky drink as a price after work." Making changes to your eating habits is still possible, indeed if you've been doing it for a longtime.Weight loss can do in the short term when drastic, abrupt adaptations are made, like only eating cabbage haze. nevertheless, similar drastic measures will not work in the long run and are neither wise nor healthy. It takes careful reflection, relief, and underpinning to change your eating habits for the long term.

Maintaining Diet

Conclusion:

We need a healthy life to make up a healthy vulnerable system and to avoid complaint. also, " maintain " means a healthy vulnerable system to cover your body. To maintain body impunity keep good habits to have regular bowel movements and normal urinary and defecation frequence, gutter bad habits, similar as smoking and heavy drinking, borrow good conduct and have regular health checks. Applicable rest exertion include walking, jogging, cycling or playing an instrument are good exertion physically and mentally. We also need to take care of our internal health since too important stress can also affect our vulnerable system. I suppose everyone needs passion in life. Because devotion means that we should do our duty to the swish. It creates one's confidence and achieved tone- achievement. These are the important element for internal health. Passion in life means we should be suitable to engage in social circumstances. healthy eating habits are essential for maintaining good health and precluding habitual conditions. Developing healthy eating habits requires making small changes to your diet and life over time. By

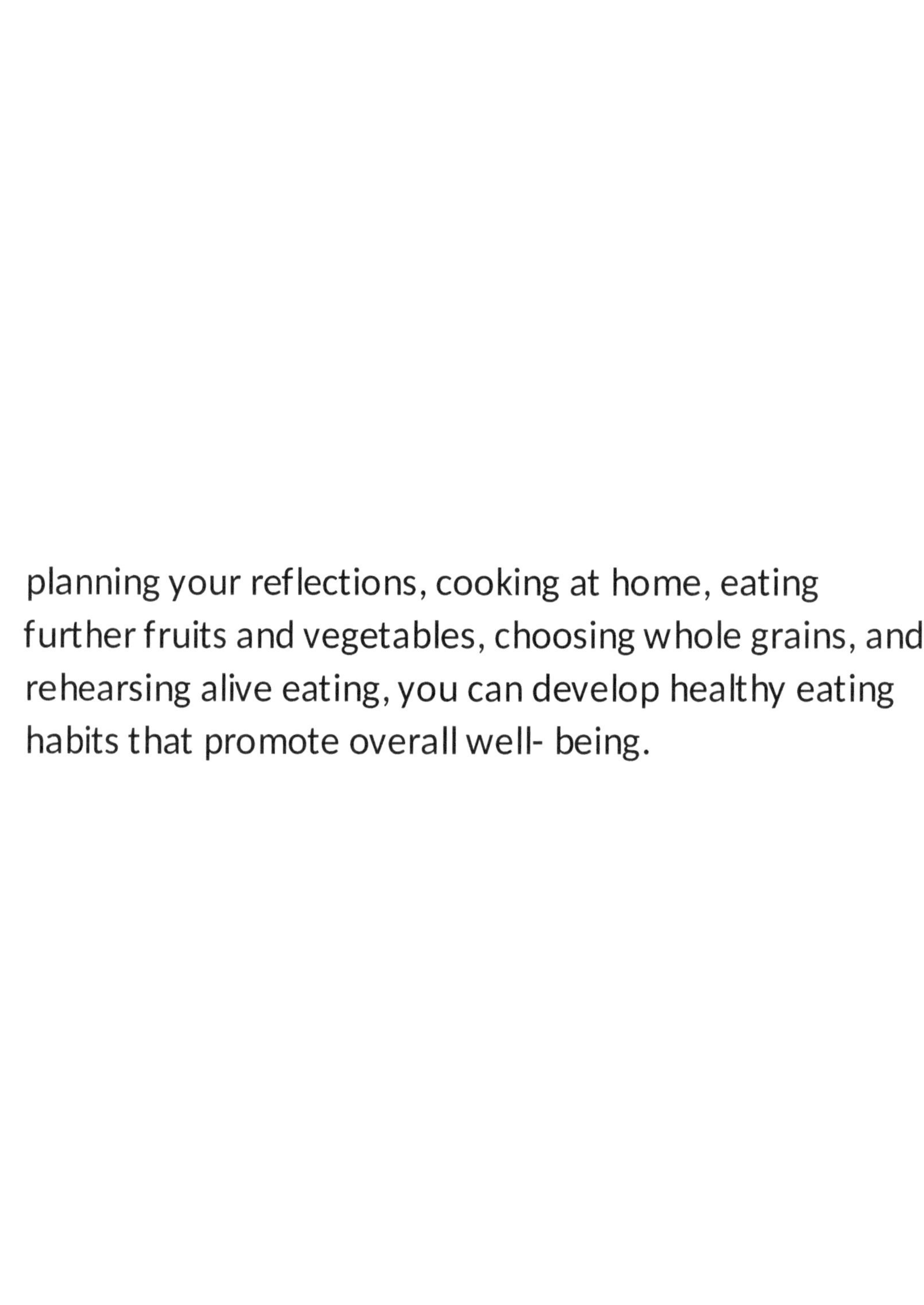

planning your reflections, cooking at home, eating further fruits and vegetables, choosing whole grains, and rehearsing alive eating, you can develop healthy eating habits that promote overall well- being.